I Love to Snort

*An Addiction Specialist's Description of
the Gradual Fall into Cocaine Addiction
and the Battle to Return to Sobriety*

Dr. Ziad Sawi MD

Contents

This book summarizes my clinical experience as I observed the subtle and gradual onset of cocaine addiction. This affliction starts in a seemingly harmless manner, initially causing few, if any, problems; however, in some patients, cocaine addiction can increasingly harm one's health, social and professional life, and family stability. Not everyone follows the same path: some people can stop cocaine use long before it becomes a serious problem, while others manage to remain as "recreational users," never progressing to habitual. The rest are not so lucky.

I've written this book in first person for dramatic effect; it is not autobiographical. Our main character is a composite of many different people I've come to know over the years. Judgmental and preachy "don't do drugs" type books are generally a boring turnoff, so it's written in a light-hearted and humorous style; however, I do not intend to mock those with serious substance use problems.

In addition to the many methods and resources available to treat cocaine and substance use disorder, I've added a guided meditation/self-hypnosis session at the end. I'm a big believer in this as a treatment – if not by itself, then in conjunction with others.

I hope readers find *I Love to Snort* both enlightening and entertaining.

Very cordially yours,

Ziad Sawi, MD

Chapter 1

The party started on a perfect note. I was with trusted friends, and we were all laughing. But I was about to be entrusted with a new secret – a rather fateful one, as things turned out.

"Do you know what would really make this party awesome?" my friend asked me. "I thought it already *was* awesome," I told him.

"Oh, you have no idea," he said with a mischievous grin. "There's a whole new level you're going to experience. I guarantee you'll love it!"

I raised my eyebrows with a Mr. Spock look of intrigue and curiosity. "Well, tell me – I'm all ears."

He motioned me to follow him. We stepped around the other party revelers and ended up...in the bathroom?

"Um...are we here for a quickie? Because I'm not really into that sort of thing..." I joked – not that there's anything wrong with that.

My friend just smiled and asked, "Wanna try some powder?" I responded with a look of bewilderment. I've been called a "witless wonder" on occasion, and probably for good reason.

"Powder? As in blow? Sugar? Nose candy? Vitamin C?"

I told you…a witless wonder...

"Cocaine??"

"Oohhhh...now I get it." I was a bit surprised but definitely curious. A bunch of thoughts ran through my head. Or maybe, in my case, slow-walked. It was like those old commercials telling me that this was my brain on drugs. But I was no prude. Plus, I had known my friend for years, and he was a responsible, stand-up guy – nothing like those TV drug fiends. He was a problem solver, the go-to guy – not some homeless junkie lying in the gutter with a needle full of heroin in his arm.

The only drug I'd ever tried was weed, and only once. I hated it, so I figured I couldn't stomach the harder stuff. Then again, everyone seemed to rave about how great cocaine was, so I figured why not; I'll try a little. I mean, what could go wrong? I wasn't the addictive type – except maybe for chocolate, candy, sugar...and, uuuhh, maybe I watched too much porn... But other than that, I definitely was not the addictive type.

I looked at my friend, and he looked at me. Then he poured a little of the white wonder on a plate and started chopping it up into a fine powder. He shaped some of it into a line, handed me a straw, and said, "Ready when you are."

As the Chinese say, "A journey of a thousand miles begins with a single step." As I soon found out, this applies to many things, not just distance. In my case, I went from trying cocaine once to a casual recreational user, then a more frequent user, until I eventually turned into a "life revolves around cocaine" user. Or should I say "substance use disorder" since the medical community feels that "addict" is a bad word.

The journey from "what harm will this do" to "my life isn't complete without it" isn't a thousand miles for everyone, though. For some, a quick walk across the street pulls them into addiction land. Some lucky ones never complete the journey: they pretty much stay in that occasional recreational user sweet spot and never have a problem. I confess that I envy them. They experience the best of both worlds – enjoying the drugs without being owned by them. Others draw the short...straw, as it were. And you never know which group you'll fall into until you roll the dice. By then, of course, it's too late.

Let me briefly step out of character and interrupt the story-telling to share some medical information about susceptibility to getting hooked on a substance.

Genetics is most definitely one of the defining factors. These days, experts have identified the specific genes closely associated with cocaine abuse, alcoholism, and other substance abuse afflictions.

The next significant factor is your age when you start using. The younger you are, the worse your chances of getting hooked. This is because your brain and neural pathways are still developing in your early 20s, and any substances you use will impact that. Just like it's easier to learn a language or pick up an instrument when you're younger, it's also easier to "learn" a drug.

And yet another crucial factor is onset speed. The quicker the drug gets you high, the more likely it will be addictive. Crack is essentially the same as cocaine, but since it's inhaled through the lungs rather than absorbed through the nasal mucosa, it ends up hitting the brain quicker, thus being much more addictive.

But now, back to our story. Where was I? Oh, yes...

My friend chopped the coke into a fine powder, shaped some into a line, and handed me the straw. (Important safety tip: in the age of COVID please don't share straws while doing coke.) I put the straw up to my right nostril, closed my left with my index finger, and just inhaled that white powder with a loud, pig-like snort.

It's difficult to look cool while doing cocaine. I mean, there you are, bent over with a straw up your nostril and closing the other like you're picking your nose while making loud snorting sounds as you inhale. Not *my* idea of sexy anyway. And yet, people do it all the time, so, I guess there's gotta be a reason.

So, after snorting a line (that word... "line" – other coke users probably consider it a tell I smile or weep when I hear it. But I digress), I straightened up, wiped my nose, and looked around. Then I looked at my friend, who was looking right back at me.

"Well, how do you feel?" he asked.

"I…don't know. How am I supposed to feel? Honestly, I don't feel that much different. I don't know why you all love this stuff so much," I replied.

"Just give it a minute," he answered back.

And so, I did. "I'm not sure. I still don't think I feel anything." But that wasn't entirely true – I was starting to feel *something*. Sure, it wasn't that magical "wow" I had seen in the movies, but it was definitely something. And it wasn't a bad something.

"Maybe I should do another line," I said. "You know, just to be sure."

And the rest, as they say, was history.

It's hard to describe the actual sensation of coke, especially to someone who's never tried it – and I'm not suggesting you do. I guess it's like a sense of happiness, of being able to handle anything. "Euphoria" is a term the medical world throws around, but I don't think it quite fits. It makes you feel very energetic, sociable, happy to be around other people and engage in conversation. Not quite euphoric, no. But people experience it a different way. Maybe euphoria *is* the right word for some, but I'll detail a better description of it later in our story.

Some people can be pretty close to normal on coke, while others can become jittery, excited, or have panic attacks. Some throw caution to the wind and take crazy risks they would usually never do, like, "If I drive twice as fast, I'll get home twice as quickly! The logic is irrefutable! What could possibly go wrong?"

Unfortunately, that pleasant sensation doesn't last forever or even for very long. After 30 minutes or so, you're kind of back to normal. Remember the old joke... "a line of cocaine makes you feel like a new man. And the first thing the new man wants is another line"?

Not all jokes are funny, but this one definitely contained some truth: it's kind of hard to do just one line. It's like you can't just eat one Pringle: before you know it, the whole cylinder is gone. Everyone can relate.

Some boring medical stuff for a moment. The American Psychiatric Association diagnoses substance use disorder (notice how they avoid "addiction," "dependence," or even "abuse") based on a set of several criteria. Number one in that set is "taking a substance in larger amounts or for a longer duration than intended."

First item on the list – check!

Then the next day comes. Experiences vary from person to person. Some friends of mine experience what's often referred to as a crash. Others feel just fine, like nothing happened. The crashers are hit with depression, anxiety, headaches, nausea, and lack of motivation. I suspect, though I'm not sure, that crashers tend to be more likely to give up cocaine earlier than non-crashers, who seemingly feel no consequences. But that's just a guess.

You've probably heard, as with many things in life, that the first time with cocaine is usually the best time. That's not entirely true. Many times after the first few, you really start to appreciate it more – an acquired taste, if you will. And the sixth or seventh time might be the best. Neuro-chemicals could be a reason for this, or it might be because cocaine quality is random. Since cocaine is an illegal substance, quality control isn't great. One batch can be much better or worse than another, so you might not experience the "good stuff" the first time. Unless you have an excellent source, your cocaine is likely mixed with all sorts of cheaper substances often more dangerous than the coke itself.

This shows the danger of "not liking cocaine too much" the first time you use it. In a way, it causes you to let down your guard. "Me? Get addicted to coke? I don't even like it that much!" Until after you've done it a few times, and then suddenly you do.

The "first time's the best time" cliché is also not entirely false: if you do coke regularly, you will start to need more and more for the same effect. Occasional users don't experience this quite as much, but the more frequent users definitely do.

Boring medical stuff: cocaine's effects are caused by the release of dopamine which then attaches to neuron receptors. Over time, your brain reduces the number of those receptors, so the dopamine has less effect. That's the mechanism behind tolerance. If you use coke more and more frequently, you experience this tolerance. And, if you find yourself needing more and more coke to get the same result, well, then congratulations! You can now check off the seventh criterion in the DSM-V list of "substance use disorder" symptoms: needing more of a substance to get the same effect. The pathway to addiction – and you aren't even trying that hard. At this rate, that journey of a thousand miles is looking more like a stroll down the street.

Chapter 2

"I never knew how awesome cocaine would be for my social life! This is the shot in the arm I've always needed!"

Over the years, the American Psychiatric Association has modified the criteria for diagnosing chemical dependence – I guess in an effort to improve it – but they always leave some gaps. Our hapless narrator is about to demonstrate one of these gaps now...

A couple of months passed since I first tried vitamin C at that party; I hadn't tried it again. It's hard to say why. I think I liked it, but it didn't wow me or anything. Besides, I had no idea where to get it. My friend was just sharing some of his stuff at that party – he wasn't dealing or anything.

But then another opportunity arose. I was at another party with a different friend who invited me to try some of his coke. Sounded good to me. This time, I could act like a man of experience instead of Mr. Witless Wonder.

And so, once again, pour the powder, chop-chop with the credit card, take the straw, and inhale. Seemed much less awkward this time, and...wow! This time it really was wow. There was a nice onset of a rush, and it kept building. Ten minutes later, double wow! The music was playing, and the moment felt perfect. Best party ever! I thought. I usually hate dancing: it burns way too many calories. But now, suddenly, it was so natural, like I was *born* to dance – or just giggle and call it dancing. Dancing, seizure disorder, whatever.

Typically a shy guy, I suddenly found it so easy to be sociable. And I don't mean obnoxious, drunk sociable, I mean self-confident and charming. People seemed to actually like talking to me. By people I mean women. I wasn't doing anything different except the vitamin C.

Cocaine! The perfect cure for introverts and hermits. Get some from your local drug dealer today! It was such an awesome moment; I simply didn't want it to end.

And it didn't have to – at least not so soon. After

an hour or so, I went to the sacred temple (AKA, the bathroom) and did another line. Damn, that stuff was some subtle magic! I found myself wishing that I had discovered cocaine sooner, as in, "Coke! Where have you been all my life?!" Cocaine had taken me from geek to super-freak in a matter of minutes. From a mere mortal at the bottom of the hill to Apollo atop Olympus. That party rolled on till the crack of dawn, and I thought I had found the Holy Grail of awesomeness. Why on earth would such a cool thing be illegal?

The demon had gotten his first claw in me, but I didn't know it at the time, and I didn't care to. I had the illusion of total control while being a puppet on a string.

I didn't want to be a freeloader. I mean, I didn't know the price of coke back then, but I knew it wasn't free – and the last thing I wanted was to be "that guy" always trying to mooch free coke. So, towards the end of the party, I approached my friend and offered to pay. Instead of taking my money, he introduced me to his "source," as they say, suggesting that I can just buy some from him and share it next time.

That seemed fair, although I hadn't ever thought of doing that; I had never bought coke before. But yeah, why not? I liked the idea of sharing. And now I could just get coke on my own instead of relying on friends. That was way more convenient. Next party was on me!

After partying all night, I went home to get some sleep. By sleep I mean lying awake, exhausted but unable to fall asleep. I wondered if the cocaine had anything to do with that. I tossed and turned for a while, then finally gave up. I walked around the house and headed to the fridge. I hadn't eaten in a long time, and I suddenly felt super hungry. I started gorging and reflecting on the previous night's events. As it turned out, I was one of the lucky ones (or unlucky, depending on how you look at it) who never experiences that post-cocaine depression or anxiety. But that lack of sleep killed me.

Fortunately, I discovered a great cure for that. Benzos! Or benzodiazepines – like Valium, or Xanax. Pop one of those after a night of heavy partying, and I slept like the dead. Hmm…bad expression, but you know what I mean…

Nattering doc interrupting again: using a second substance to counteract the unwanted side effects of the first substance is not on the DSM-V list – but it's definitely a sign IMHO.

...Sunday was recovery day, and by nighttime, I had no trouble sleeping. I woke up on Monday morning, ready for work and feeling very upbeat about the new changes in my life.

Something had definitely changed. I wasn't sure what it was at the time, but I knew something was different. In retrospect, I now know exactly what it was: the first thing was priorities. My priority became the next weekend and the next chance to party. Then, with the contact my friend gave me, I no longer had to wait until someone else threw one. I could be the host.

And so, another barrier was broken: I had my own source. He was really a friend of my friend's friend, but still, I had the direct line. I sent a text to the number I was given and got a reply fifteen minutes later. Long story short, we ended up meeting in a parking lot for the exchange. I bought a decent amount because, as with anything else, cocaine is cheaper in bulk. Makes good financial sense, you know. I had also been told that you never know when your source would run dry, so I figured I'd better have some for a rainy day.

Boring medical stuff: Notice how our hapless character is more and more engrossed in the hunt for cocaine. Check off another in the DSM-V list of symptoms: more time spent using or trying to obtain the substance. Now, back to our character…

The second thing that changed, perhaps something I didn't notice at the time, was a subtle division among my friends. I subconsciously split them up into the cocaine group – the ones I loved partying with – and those I now dubbed as my "vanilla friends": the ones who could never know about my new lifestyle. I found myself avoiding them; they just weren't much fun. Still, at the time, I either didn't notice, or I just didn't give it a thought, like it was the most natural thing to do, done automatically.

Boring doctor stuff: what our hapless character describes is not exactly on the DSM-V list of symptoms. They mention social, interpersonal problems related to use, although I don't think our character is quite there yet. Still, definitely be on the lookout for rearranging social commitments if you happen to be traveling down this path.

Chapter 3

"I never really drank much until I started doing cocaine."

The week would fly by and the weekend would come, where I could now be the cool party dude – the one with all the special refreshments taking the event to a whole new level. I was building a rep! Life seemed good. But, of course, I was gradually reorienting that life to revolve around that precious vitamin C, always planning parties and looking for new people into the same lifestyle as me. Now spending less and less time with those boring vanilla friends.

In many ways, substance use – cocaine or any other – is a kind of exploration, where discovering new and innovative ways to use your drug of choice is part of the journey. One of the early discoveries I and probably many other snorters made was how differently we looked at alcohol. As previously mentioned, everyone will react differently. For certain people, mixing alcohol and coke will make them as sick as a homeless dog. Others are fine. Of course, both groups love the combination while they're in the moment; it's the next day or later that night when the truth will be revealed. Although too late, of course, leaving many hungover souls to wonder what they were thinking. As with many missteps in life, you can file this one under "it seemed like a good idea at the time."

Fortunately (or not), I was among the group that didn't have any such problem. Combining the two creates a whole new level of fun and games. *Now* you could call it euphoria, and I would agree. It also makes the cocaine sensation last longer, and since alcohol is cheaper and easier to come by than cocaine, it's quite a bargain and time-saver. With that discovery, I started drinking more. And more. And the parties became better and better. With such a neat little combination, everything seemed grand, and life was good. What could possibly go wrong?

Let me pause the narration for some more boring medical stuff.

1. Cocaine combined with alcohol is several times more dangerous than either one by itself.

Keep in mind that alcohol on its own is probably more toxic than cocaine. Don't be fooled just because one is legal and the other isn't; laws are often pretty random.

2.   When then two are combined, your body creates a substance called cocaethylene. CE is very toxic to your heart. Over time, it will catch up with you. I'm not one to judge or moralize, but keep it in mind.

3.   Combining alcohol and cocaine triggers dopamine release, which is why people like doing it. However, they cause the release using different pathways, thus releasing even more of that super-fun dopamine. And since cocaine is a stimulant while alcohol is a depressant, they often blunt one another's side effects. You can drink a lot more alcohol when you're doing cocaine, and you won't even notice you're drunk – but trust me, you are. Without the coke, you would have passed out several drinks ago. With it, you're the Energizer Bunny of alcohol – and alcohol toxicity can easily go unnoticed.

4.   The reverse is also true. Cocaine might make people jittery, give them a racing heart, or make them feel a little stressed. But washing it down with a couple of shots of your drink of choice really takes the edge off and saves the day. Or so it seems.

This is why the two, coke and alcohol, seem a match made in heaven to some. I'm not here to browbeat, point fingers, or *tsk tsk* anyone; I only wish to inform and hopefully entertain.

And now, back to our character.

I was loving life at this point. I was all about parties and hanging out with like-minded friends – the more the merrier. I did, however, begin to notice a *feeew* minor drawbacks. I would say I have a pretty strong constitution, I work out, and I rarely get sick. But I started to experience something new for me: hangovers. Not severe, but definitely noticeable, especially to someone like me who was feeling pretty invincible at that point.

Was it the coke? Noooo, cocaine is my friend. He loves me. It was probably the alcohol. Well, indirectly, the coke. The thing is, it's really easy to lose track of how much you're drinking with cocaine. Have I done three shots? Or is it six now? Whatever, I can do one more. How many is it now? Never mind, I'm feeling pretty groovy, and the party's just getting started.

Instead of shots, I started mixing vodka with a little soda to make it more tolerable – one shot per glass. Except…I was kind of *gestalting* it, pouring what I thought was one shot into the glass (which was a pretty tall glass, by the way) and then tipping some soda

over it. But I measured it the next day and what I thought was one shot was actually about three – so, I was drinking three times more alcohol than I thought I had. Maybe more or even much more because, as I mentioned, I kind of lost track of how many glasses I'd had.

Now that I think about it, it was a miracle the hangovers weren't way worse. Thank heaven for small favors, I guess.

All this led me to the other new phenomenon I noticed: blackouts. Has someone ever told you some crazy thing you did at a party, but you have absolutely no memory of it? It's definitely disconcerting the first time it happens, especially when they describe what you did and it's something you simply would never, ever do. I'm going to skip the details here, but trust me – it ain't pretty.

Forgive me for interrupting, but dull doctor stuff again: we mentioned using a substance in greater amounts than intended as a DSM-V symptom. Losing track of how much you've actually used is not on the list, but it is definitely a warning sign. Granted, our character is referring to alcohol, but I wouldn't be surprised if he'd also lost track of how many lines he's done…

…Still, I was feeling good about everything overall. Yeah, the occasional hangover was bad, but like I said, some people really get hammered when they mix coke and alcohol. Others have a fantastic time with the combination, doing shot after shot interspersed with line after line. One moment they're on top of the world, and the next, it's like a near-death experience – like being struck by lightning from a clear blue sky. They would suddenly feel horribly sick, weak, miserable, and dehydrated, with toxic amounts of alcohol in their body. That usually meant others would gather around for reassurance (because they really felt like they were going to die) and rehydration. Hopefully, they could drink water without throwing up. You're very sympathetic at first, but when the same people do the same thing party after party, it starts to get pretty old. I would have to stop inviting them. You know, for their own good. And mine.

But, those severe attacks never happened to me, so I was all right. No problems here. Let the games begin!

Chapter 4

"I've started to notice some strange things happening."

So far, I've been describing party times, always on weekends and holidays. What was I up to the rest of the week? Well, I went to work as always. No problems of any kind, on time every time, never called in sick, missed a deadline, or did substandard work. Cocaine and partying were just for the weekends – workdays were kept totally separate.

...Until they weren't. Because here's the tricky part: if you can keep the snorting to just once in a while, only-on-weekends kind of thing, you'll probably be okay. I don't recommend it, but some people can definitely do that. You just never know if you're one of them until you roll the dice. By then, of course, it's too late.

For me, party days and workdays were separate for quite a while. But keeping them separate proved to be easier said than done. The pattern went like this: I figured that if one weekend a month was fun, then two would be twice as nice. And then, well, why not three? I mean, as long as it's only weekends and never on work nights... As long as I had the next day to mope around the house while recovering, then there should really be no problem.

Nagging doctor again: did we talk about more and more time spent using? I think we did. I'm sure we mentioned more time spent obtaining the substance, which is closely related. Back to our character...

...As long as I didn't have to work the next day, everything would be okay – as long as I didn't cross the line.

That evil word, "line." As in, "stay in line." As in, "walk the line." As in, "let's do another line!" That word will always have a completely different meaning for me. Closing my eyes and thinking, "Let's do another line" will forever remind me of Dorothy closing her eyes and saying, "There's no place like home." (Spot of trivia! Judy Garland suffered from alcoholism, cocaine, and barbiturate use disorder. Tragically, she died by suicide).

One Tuesday, a couple of friends (not of the vanilla kind, if you get my drift) called up and asked if they could stop by for a little while. Me being me, always wanting to be the good host and feeling kind of bored, I figured I wouldn't mind some company.

I was thinking, "I really have to work tomorrow," but somehow my mouth said, "Sure guys, come on over." Not sure how it happened. I did catch myself and said that I couldn't stay up too late as I had work the next day.

"Oh, sure," they said. "Just a little while. I found a great new source! You really have to try this." Danger, Will Robinson, danger!

"We'll just do a line or two, that's all…" It's a trap!

Two key phrases stick out. The first is "a great new source." At that time, we all were always on the lookout for purer and better cocaine. It became a kind of competition. And whenever one of us scored a really good batch, we naturally wanted to show off. We all wanted to achieve that cocaine Zen status and be the guy (or gal, as the case may be) with the great hookup.

I'm sure you've guessed the other key phrase: "just one or two lines." If it really were that easy to stop at one or two, then no one would be a coke addict. Just like if it were that easy to stop at just one Pringle, no one would be fat.

But, of course, we often have to learn the hard way. And so, I thought, "Well, if it's just one or two lines..." And a moment later, my friends were at the door.

It really was a good batch. Of course, mixing it with alcohol made it even better, plus the company of fun friends. It was such a great combination that no one except a party pooper would want to stop too early. And no one ever wants to be the party pooper, the wimp who's the first to say goodnight – especially when everyone's having such a good time... So good a time that it was easy to forget I had to work the next day.

Another key phrase I repeatedly heard that night: "Okay, just one last line."

And so, the party went on. And on. And on. Ten PM suddenly became one AM, then four...and then five… Kind of close to getting up for work. It was about then that the brief "just one or two lines" party came to an end.

I had an hour to sleep. But who was I kidding? There was no way I was going to fall asleep. I essentially had an hour to lay in bed and think about how stupid I had been and how hellishly exhausted I was, wondering how the hell I was going to get through a whole day of work. At what point did this seem like a good idea? At what point did I lose control and cross the line? As in, "let's do another line!"

Suddenly, I found the answer. Well, it seemed like the answer at the time. Maybe it wasn't the best answer. Maybe it was downright stupid, but it seemed like the least bad option. Calling in sick was a no-no: I had never done it, and I definitely didn't want to start. I had a rep as being Mr. Reliable, the go-to guy. I couldn't throw that away. I was the problem solver; I didn't want to become the problem.

So, I got out of bed and walked downstairs. I looked at the plate of cocaine and used my credit card to scrape up the last few flakes. As was often the case, there was actually quite a bit of cocaine there – enough for a nice, juicy, fat line. I took that hit through the nose, and some sweet energy started coursing its way through me. I could make it through the day. I wasn't happy with myself, but hey! I didn't call in sick. That's one line I'd never cross.

Goddamn it, I was still okay.

Me, the nattering doc again: using the substance in hazardous conditions fulfills yet another of the DSM-V list of symptoms...

Chapter 5

"That Pavlov dude really knew what he was talking about!"

And I bet he wasn't only talking about dogs. I'm sure you've all heard of Pavlov's experiment in conditioning, where dogs learned to salivate when they heard the bell ring and thought it was feeding time. Actually, they reacted to seeing the white lab coats, but never mind.

Humans can be conditioned just as easily as dogs, and that includes people who like cocaine. So many environmental triggers can get a cocaine user to think about and react to cocaine. Pavlov seemed so insightful that I almost wondered if he was a coke fiend. (To the best of myknowledge, he was not, and I imagine it would have been rather hard to find a good source living in the early days of the Soviet Union).

Back to our story…

…I noticed that, even during sober periods, it was

very easy for something to trigger thoughts of cocaine. Scrolling through Netflix, it seemed like every other movie reminded me of it. I viewed Narcos from a very different perspective. It just felt different to me than it probably did to others. Watching that scene in Pulp Fiction with Uma Thurman in the bathroom simply made me say Goddamn! And then smile with that mischievous smile. It was like listening to a hilarious joke that no one got except you.

But it did present a problem: when I wasn't doing cocaine, I was *thinking* about cocaine. Out of sight, out of mind, they say, but it was never actually out of sight. Something always reminded me. And that was just movies. Ever listen to music and notice how many songs are about cocaine? I sure have. And no matter what, I would see or hear something that made coke run all the way from the back of my mind to the first aforethought.

Boring medical stuff: there's an observed phenomenon among heavy substance users (cocaine, alcohol, etc.) in which everyday events trigger thoughts of their drug of choice.

With alcoholics, for example, watching someone pour something into a glass reminds them of drinking when they're sober, eliciting cravings and making it that much harder to quit. Oh, cravings! That's another symptom on that DSM-V list.

Chapter 6

"Even paranoids have enemies."

Back to our story…

So, you've divided your life into two separate (more or less) parts. One is your crazy, coked-up nightlife, and the other is your straight-laced, responsible worker, family, vanilla friends life. If the second group consists of people who would really frown upon your wild side, then you really have to keep that part under wraps. The barrier separating your two sides has to be a tall stone wall. It's not hard to do at first. After a while, though, you begin to wonder... Am I behaving differently? Do they suspect? My God, what will I do if everyone finds out? You start to wonder if everything is still the same. Am I slipping up at work? Do I look as exhausted as I feel? Do people think I'm withdrawn? Absent and in a daze? Am I making mistakes? Forgetting things I was supposed to do? "Hey, what's that white powder under your nose?" A question much easier to ask than to answer. You worry if they *did* notice it, and if they did, how quickly would your whole world crash down around you.

It wasn't a problem in the beginning. But then, as you may assume, things progress.

If you don't happen to be particularly wealthy, one thing that might prove awkward is that cocaine is not exactly cheap. I mean, it's cheap enough if you only do it every now and again, but once it becomes an all-the-time thing, the costs add up pretty fast. If you live alone, you can kind of get by for a while longer. But if you have a family to support, then they will start to notice when money gets tight – because money for cocaine has to come from somewhere, like the money that's wasted on, oh, I dunno…bills and rent and such frivolous things. It becomes hard to hide that from the wife, especially when they expect silly things like gifts on their birthday or anniversary or Christmas.

Fortunately, I never had that problem, but I know many who have. Suddenly, the wife's credit card isn't working (maxed out, of course. Hard to explain that one) and secrets kept in the dark are now out in bright sunlight.

So, how do you avoid that problem? Well, you can start earning extra money on the side by...dealing coke. Multiple streams of income! Coke now no longer breaks the bank but actually helps pay the bills. Nice guy, that Cocaine. But that's a story for another day.

Chapter 7

"Cocaine the...gateway drug?"

Opponents of marijuana often call it the gateway drug: the softer substance that invariably leads to the harder ones. In our character's case, that doesn't describe it at all...

...I tried marijuana years before I ever tasted coke, and I hated it. I didn't bother with any other drug for years, either. If anything, my experience with weed acted as a mental barrier, stopping me from trying anything stronger.

Then along came cocaine, and with it the irresistible urge to experiment. I discussed the coke and alcohol combination earlier, but why stop there, I figured? And so, at another party at the suggestion of another friend, I tried some more weed immediately after a line of coke.

Strangely, surprisingly, wildly...it was much better than I remembered it. In fact, it was pretty awesome.

Oddly enough, cocaine was my gateway drug that opened the way to marijuana, which I had always hated...until I combined it with cocaine, exactly the opposite of what you might expect. Each affects the brain differently – kind of like a pro wrestling tag team, with each wrestler pulling a different cool move in your mind.

That's when I decided to become a scientist of sorts, conducting wild and crazy new experiments. An explorer/adventurer seeking out new places and experiences. It was all for science, after all.

And so, in my scientific mind, I thought – quite logically, of course – that if cocaine plus alcohol is good and cocaine plus weed is good, then what would it be like to combine all three? The scientific community needed an answer, and I was just the man to get it! Explorer and adventurer that I was, I decided on the best environment for such an experiment. Time for another party!

Long story short, everyone had a great time, and I experienced new dimensions of neurochemical craziness.

But why stop there? Since that experiment was a great success, let's try another one – such as cocaine plus an opiate. These days, everyone has a friend of a friend with some Percocet or norco. Cocaine plus opiates? Good! Cocaine plus opiates plus alcohol? Very, very good! Cocaine plus opiates plus alcohol plus weed? Freaking genius! Cocaine plus opiates, plus weed plus alcohol plus ecstasy? Fucking Nobel Prize in chemistry! I had no idea I had such a talent for science.

But…the day after such experiments, the lab, otherwise known as my brain, was an absolute mess. In other words, even the toughest of drug fiends will get the most devastating of hangovers when you get to this new level of crazy. And those hangovers lasted a *loooong* time.Way longer than the fun part.

Doctor stuff again: one substance leading to the use of others is not among the DSM-V symptoms, but it is a huge sign that things are getting way out of hand.

Chapter 8

"Slowly, slowly...then all of a sudden…"

Back to our character...

…Yes, the hangover often lasted longer than the fun part, but the fun part was oh so much fun! So much fun that, despite all the subsequent pain I *knew* was coming, I just kept on doing it anyway. The last time I did, it was undoubtedly the best. It was a party that just would not stop, should not, could not stop. And for an extraordinarily long time, it did not stop.

It was a Saturday at my place. Everyone was invited, and everyone showed up. It was wall-to-wall action with music, alcohol, cocaine, ecstasy, and all and sundry. A couple of my vanilla friends who had heard about these Great Gatsby-like events I was rumored to host demanded they be invited. I loved that reputation! It made me feel oh-so gangster!

But one has to be careful with these things. I had to make sure these vanilla friends could safely enter the world of bright colors and that they could be entrusted with our secret. Snitches and tattletales were the last things I needed. But they were persistent.

"Okay," I told them. "Come by at eight, prepare to stay late, and keep an open mind." They all agreed, and with great excitement, they all showed up right on the dot: no effort to be fashionably late.

A few awkward moments passed – you know, when there's a big event but only a few people show up at the very start? But that didn't last as more and more people started rolling in. Soon, the perfect crowd was in the house, and the atmosphere was electric. Of course, as the party progressed, everyone headed to the secret temple – the bathroom – with the cocaine. Mind you, almost everyone at the party was in the know – only a handful of vanilla friends were in attendance, but they did notice people would disappear and then reappear in a delightful state of mind.

"What's going on?" they asked me. "Are you sure you guys want to know?"

"Definitely! Don't keep secrets from us – we've been your friends for years! Quit being so...aloof."

Aloof...they were unaware that they had been downgraded to mere vanilla friends. Far too boring for my new, super-exciting lifestyle. But I knew I was being unfair; they were good people and had been my friends in need on more than one occasion. They deserved better than how I had been treating them. The least I could do was pay it forward.

So, what better way to make things up to them than by introducing them to cocaine? It seemed to change my life for the better, or so I thought (remember, witless wonder…).

"Well, far be it from me to be aloof. I wanna be the good buddy by your side. So, if you guys are ready…" They seemed to hang on to my every word, like they were watching a Game of Thrones or Walking Dead season cliffhanger. Hmm…given the environment, let's go with the TWD analogy.

"Have you guys ever tried vitamin C?" "Huh?" they asked in unison.

"As in powder? Sugar? Nose candy? Vitamin C?!"

Deer in the headlights. I mean, come on, how clueless can you be?"Cocaine?'"

A ghost must have passed them from the way their jaws dropped.

"Wow! Is that what's been different about you? We would never have guessed."

"Wanna try some?"

They were very hesitant but curious at the same time.

"Just a little taste. If you don't like it, no need to try more."

As you can imagine, most people like it.

It didn't take much convincing before they were ready to give it a try. And so, I led them to the secret temple and introduced them to my cool druggie friends, each offering warm greetings and encouragement. My (formerly) vanilla friends felt very much at home.

As the past, so the future. I broke off a nice, rocky piece (of course, I made sure I had some very pure powder that night – my vanilla friends deserved the best) and crushed it with the flat side of a credit card, *chop chop chop*, to form it into a few lines (remember that word? It never gets old). With one line for each new inductee into our circle, I handed them each a short straw (a clean straw...COVID and all), and the rest, as they say, is history.

I think my new friends had the most fabulous time of their lives. They were quick to discover the alcohol plus cocaine witches' brew, and they really loved it. I actually had to pretend to be responsible and hold them back before they overdid it – because, believe me, the tendency is to overdo it.

Just like that, my vanilla friends joined my inner circle of druggie friends. And all lived happily ever after.

Boring doctor stuff: getting a thrill out of introducing a substance to newbies isn't one of the infamous symptoms, but it's a sign.

...And here is where I cut my story short. The paths ahead are variable. All the post-party headaches could lead some people to pull back from the edge before it's too late. Others just keep getting sucked in deeper and deeper. For some, there is no such thing as rock bottom. Just a bottomless pit, and you keep on falling. You can use your imagination – I won't moralize.

But things like oversleeping, missing work, and failure to be there for family, are the sorts of things you can expect on the way down.

Which group will you fall into? Until you start down that road, you can't know. By then, of course, it's too late.

Lastly, I leave you with this self-guided meditation/hypnosis session. I firmly believe regular meditation sessions will help in recovering from substance use. It's best in conjunction withother treatments, but I believe that it's still useful by itself.

Hypnosis/Guided Meditation

Script for recovery from cocaine addiction

Sit in a comfortable chair or lie down in a comfortable bed. Ensure that your back is supported by the chair's back, a cushion, or a pillow. Now that you are in a comfortable posture, I want you to select some point or something in your room to look at. While looking make sure that your neck and eyes are at ease and comfortable. Now begin to focus on that point or location that you have chosen. Keep looking… Keep looking… Now the more you look, you will start to feel this sensation of heaviness in your eyes. This feeling of heaviness is starting to increase and your eyes are getting heavy. The more you look the heavier your eyes will get. You will notice that your breathing is getting heavy and deep. Now because of this sense of heaviness in your eyes, you are having this strong urge to blink. Now blink slowly and gently. Blink again… Now slowly close your eyes. Take a deep slow gentle breath. Breathe in fully and deeply.

Breathe out slowly and fully. Once again breathe in and breathe out.

Now put one hand on your heart and another hand on your belly. Now as you breathe in and breathe out pay attention to how your belly moves up and down. Now as you continue to breathe in and breathe out, bring your attention to the rhythmic beating of your heart. Notice the pace of rhythmic breathing of your heart. Now I am going to count from 10 down to zero and as I count from 10 down to zero, your body and mind will start to get deeply relaxed and you will go into the state of deep deep relaxation. 10..9..8..7..6..5..4..3..2..1. **(Snaps fingers).**

Now DEEP SLEEP.

Now imagine yourself walking by the beautiful beach on a cool windy evening. You notice the deep blue water of the beach. You notice how rhythmically and aesthetically waves of water are flowing with each other. This serene sight of deep blue water will fill you with a sense of purity. Your body and mind are feeling calm and in harmony. Now you slowly walk towards this deep blue water and gently put your one foot in the water. You feel this sense of coolness and deep relaxation running through your foot towards your whole body. You are feeling light, refreshed, energized, and rejuvenated. Take few moments to let those feelings of lightness, calmness, freedom flow through your mind and body. Now take a slow walk on the cool sand. Feel the soft coolness of sand and the feeling of liberation flowing through your body and mind. Take your time **(pause- for 5 seconds)**, now when you are ready say to yourself:

I love myself. I respect myself. I am a brave and confident person. I believe in myself. I am in control. I am the master of my thoughts and cravings. I am stronger than my cravings. I do not give up easily. I am getting stronger every day mentally and physically. I am a strong, powerful person who has strong willpower. I am becoming a better and best version of myself every day. I am in control of my impulses. I deserve a good life. I am capable of achieving my best self and my target goals. My possibilities are limitless. Nothing can stop me. I am capable of dealing with any difficulty that comes in the way of maintaining my sobriety. My past has no power over me. I let go of my past. I forgive myself for the habit of addiction. I know it is okay to make mistakes and I forgive myself for making the mistakes during the habit of addiction. I am free from every shackle now. Any kind of addiction has no control over me. I am in charge of my emotions, and my actions. External events have no power over me. Nothing can upset me until I permit it to do so. I am doing great. I am a powerful person who is motivated and driven to choose sobriety. I am unstoppable in achieving anything I want to that benefits me, my present, and my future. I am making a good life for myself. I am a future-oriented person. I am working every day on myself and on my goals to be my optimal self. I make my future. I believe in myself and my abilities. My physical and mental health are my top priorities. I am at peace. I am calm. I am safe. I am worthy. I am enough. I deserve a good life. I have the power to change my story and turn around my life the way I want my life to be. I am a courageous person who can say "no". I establish healthy boundaries. I deserve to be happy. I am proud of myself to be on the right path. I am a conscious person. I choose to be positive, optimistic. I chose to live intentionally and fearlessly. I am free of any mental resistance. I choose my well-being over everything.

Now take a deep breath. Bring your attention to the rhythmic beating of your heart. Bring a feeling of gratitude towards your body. Think about how grateful and blessed you are to be in a command of a healthy body. Now take few moments to feel gratitude.

Now bring your attention back to the current moment. Take a deep breath in and out. Take a deep breath in through your nose and out through your mouth. Inhale deeply and exhale deeply once more. Now I am going to count down from ten to one. And as I count... you will gradually become more aware, returning to the present time, and will slowly start to open your eyes. 10... 9...8...7...6...5...4...3...2... and 1. Start to stretch slowly and avoid making any sudden movements. Gently and slowly open your eyes, feeling calm, free, positive, peaceful, liberated, motivated, confident, and alert.